CAVE WRAPS

40 FAST & EASY PALEO RECIPES
FOR THE BEST DAMN WRAPS EVER

PRINTED IN THE UNITED STATES OF AMERICA

FIRST PRINTING, 2013

ISBN-13:
978-0615805375
ISBN-10:
061580537X

SALEM FOX PRESS

WWW.SALEMFOX.COM

CONTENTS

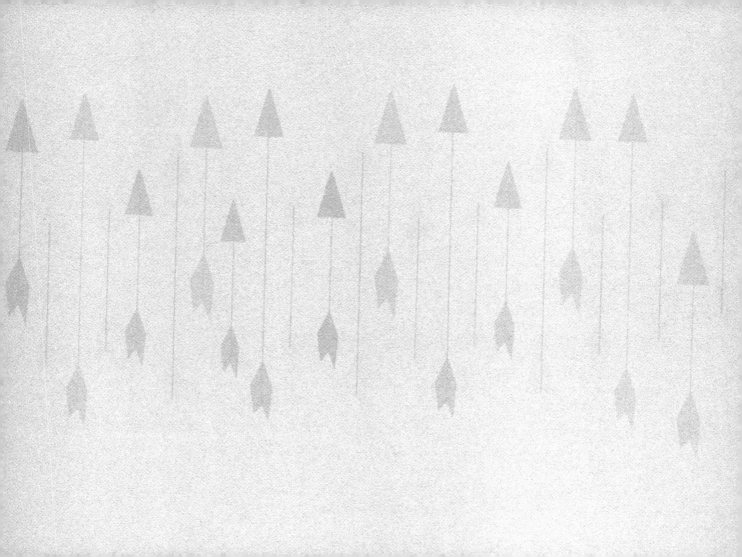

FAQ

HOW MANY SLICES OF MEAT DO YOU USE TO MAKE A WRAP?

IN THE RECIPES, WE CALL FOR 1 THICK SLICE OF MEAT. HOWEVER, THE THICKNESS AND LENGTH OF EACH SLICE OF MEAT WILL VARY, AND IN MANY OF THE PHOTOS, YOU CAN SEE THAT IT TOOK ANYWHERE FROM 1-3 SLICES OF MEAT TO CREATE THE WRAP. YES, WE CHEATED! SOMETIMES WE LIKE TO CREATE WRAPS WITH DOUBLE OR TRIPLE THE MEAT, JUST TO MAKE IT MORE FILLING.

WHAT ARE THE BLUE SPHERES I SEE ON SOME OF YOUR WRAPS?

THOSE ARE DECORATIVE TOOTHPICKS! SOMETIMES THESE WRAPS JUST WON'T STAY CLOSED, AND AT THOSE TIMES, WE PULL OUT OUR TRUSTY TOOTHPICKS.

MANY OF YOUR RECIPES CALL FOR SALSA OR GUACAMOLE. WHAT ARE SOME GOOD PALEO RECIPES FOR THOSE?

WE BELIEVE IN KEEPING SALSA AND GUACAMOLE AS SIMPLE AS POSSIBLE. TURN THE PAGE FOR THE RECIPES WE USE TO CREATE DELICIOUS PALEO GUACAMOLE AND SALSA.

PALEO SALSA

INGREDIENTS:
4 TOMATOES, DICED
1/3 CUP ONIONS, CHOPPED
2 TABLESPOONS CILANTRO, CHOPPED
2 TABLESPOONS GREEN CHILIS
1/2 JALAPENO, MINCED
1 TABLESPOON LIME JUICE
1 TEASPOON GARLIC, MINCED
1/2 TEASPOON SALT
1/2 TEASPOON CUMIN

DIRECTIONS:
MIX IT ALL TOGETHER IN A BOWL.

THIS SALSA TASTES AMAZING FRESH, BUT IT'S
EVEN BETTER AFTER SITTING IN YOUR
REFRIGERATOR FOR A COUPLE OF DAYS.

PALEO GUACAMOLE

INGREDIENTS:
1/2 CUP PALEO SALSA
2 AVOCADOS

DIRECTIONS:
MASH UP THE AVOCADOS AND MIX IN THE SALSA

TO KEEP THE GUACAMOLE GREEN AND FRESH
FOR SEVERAL DAYS, PLACE PLASTIC WRAP OVER
THE GUACAMOLE, SO THAT IT'S TOUCHING THE
GUACAMOLE, AND SEAL THE BOWL WITH THE
PLASTIC WRAP AS TIGHTLY AS POSSIBLE. IT'S
IMPORTANT THAT THE PLASTIC WRAP BE
PRESSED COMPLETELY AGAINST THE GUACA-
MOLE, MAKING IT AS AIR-TIGHT AS POSSIBLE!

I'M SORRY, BUT SOME OF THESE AREN'T REALLY RECIPES. THEY'RE JUST A FEW INGREDIENTS SHOVED INTO A MEAT WRAP! WHAT GIVES?

THE GOAL WHEN CREATING CAVE WRAPS WAS TO CREATE DELICIOUS WRAPS THAT ARE FAST AND EASY TO MAKE. WE WEREN'T TRYING TO MAKE ANYTHING GOURMET OR COMPLICATED. WHAT WE WERE TRYING TO CREATE IS A BOOK THAT SHOWS YOU HOW TO CREATE MEALS THAT ARE:

* INCREDIBLY TASTY
* SOMETHING YOU MAY NEVER THOUGHT OF BEFORE
* EASY TO WHIP UP IN A FEW MINUTES
* PALEO

CAVE WRAPS ARE FOR REAL PEOPLE WITH BUSY LIVES WHO WANT TO EAT SOMETHING NUTRITIOUS AND SERIOUSLY TASTY, BUT DON'T HAVE TIME TO MAKE HOMEMADE MAYO OR SCOUR STORES FOR PALEO-FRIENDLY BREAD ALTERNATIVES. ALL THE PALEO WRAPS IN CAVE WRAPS USE INCREDIBLY EASY TO FIND, COMMON INGREDIENTS AND THEY'RE SIMPLE TO CREATE.

WHY ARE THE MEAT SLICES IN SOME OF YOUR CAVE WRAPS HEATED AND OTHERS NOT?

WE LIKE TO MIX IT UP! WE ALSO JUST WANTED TO SHOW YOU THAT MANY WRAPS CAN BE MADE WITHOUT TURNING ON THE STOVE AND MANY WRAPS TASTE JUST AS GOOD COLD AS THEY DO HOT. NONE OF THE WRAPS REQUIRE THE MEAT SLICES TO BE HEATED, IT JUST TASTES BETTER THAT WAY SOMETIMES. HEAT THEM UP OR EAT THEM COLD, THEY'RE YUMMY EITHER WAY!

4

WHY ARE THERE NO SERVING SIZES INCLUDED IN YOUR RECIPES?

EACH RECIPE ASSUMES YOU WILL CREATE ONE WRAP. IF YOU WANT MORE THAN ONE WRAP, JUST MULTIPLY THE INGREDIENTS TO CREATE THE AMOUNT OF WRAPS YOU NEED.

WHY DON'T YOUR RECIPES CALL FOR ORGANIC INGREDIENTS OR GRASS-FED MEAT?

WHEN WE CREATED THE WRAPS FOR CAVE WRAPS, WE ONLY USED ORGANIC PRODUCE AND THE HIGHEST QUALITY MEAT. HOWEVER, YOU'RE FREE TO USE WHATEVER PRODUCE AND MEAT YOU LIKE. INSTEAD OF WRITING THE WORD "ORGANIC" IN FRONT OF EACH INGREDIENT, WE ASSUME YOU'LL JUST GO AHEAD AND BUY ORGANIC IF THAT'S YOUR THING.

WHEN ARE WE GOING TO GET TO THE WRAPS?
RIGHT NOW! ON TO THE WRAPS!

TURKEY

APPLE FESTIVAL TURKEY WRAP

Ingredients

* 1 Small Apple, Diced
* 1/3 Cup Applesauce
* 2 Tablespoons Cashews
* Thick Cut Slice of Turkey

Directions

1. Heat the turkey slice on pan or over a panini grill.

2. Stuff the turkey slice with apples, applesauce, and cashews.

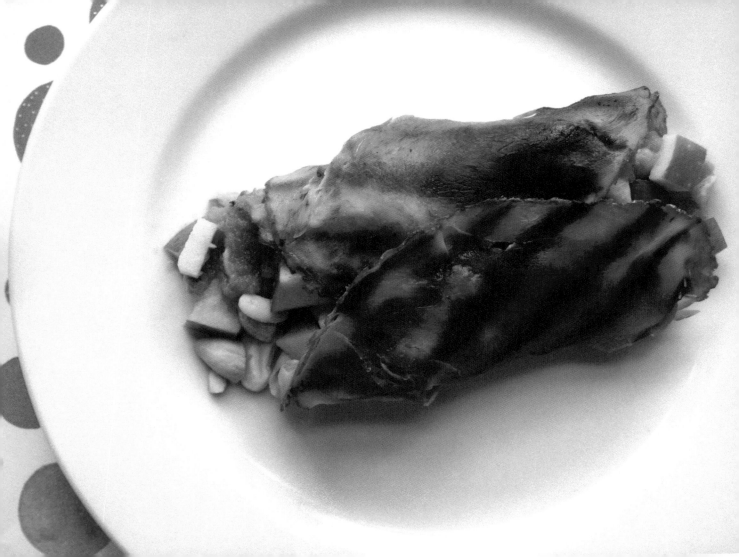

BERRY NUTTY TURKEY WRAP

Ingredients

* 1/3 Cup Strawberries, Sliced
* 1/3 Cup Blueberries
* 1/3 Cup Blackberries
* 2 Tablespoons Cashews
* 1/3 Cup Arugula
* Thick Cut Slice of Turkey

Directions

1. Heat the turkey slice on pan or over a panini grill.

2. Stuff the turkey slice with berries, cashews, and arugula.

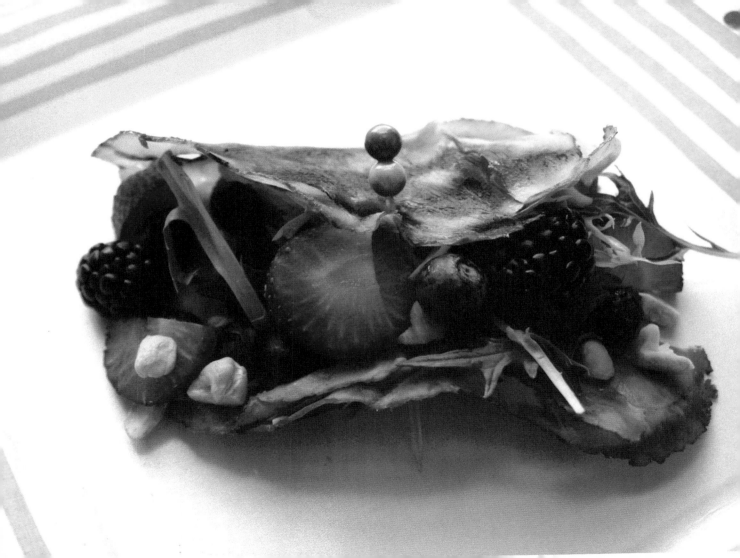

CHICKEN BACON TURKEY WRAP

Ingredients

* 2 Slices Thin Cut Chicken, Thawed
* 1 Teaspoon Olive Oil
* 2 Bacon Slices, Cooked
* 3 Tablespoons Guacamole
* 1/4 Bell Pepper, Sliced
* 1/4 Cup Cucumber, Sliced
* Thick Cut Slice of Turkey

Directions

1. Heat the thin cut chicken and oil over medium heat until cooked through.

2. Heat the turkey slice on pan or over a panini grill.

3. Stuff the turkey slice with bacon, guacamole, peppers, and cucumber.

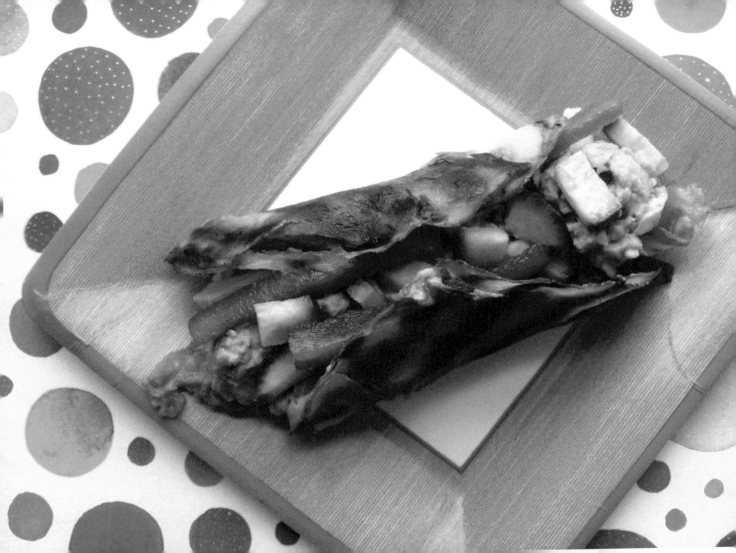

TUNA & PINEAPPLE TURKEY WRAP

Ingredients

* 1 Can Tuna
* 1/2 Cup Pineapple
* 1/3 Cup Salsa
* 1/4 Cup Celery, Sliced
* Thick Cut Slice of Turkey

Directions

1. Mix tuna, pineapple, salsa, and celery in a bowl.

2. Stuff turkey slice with tuna mixture.

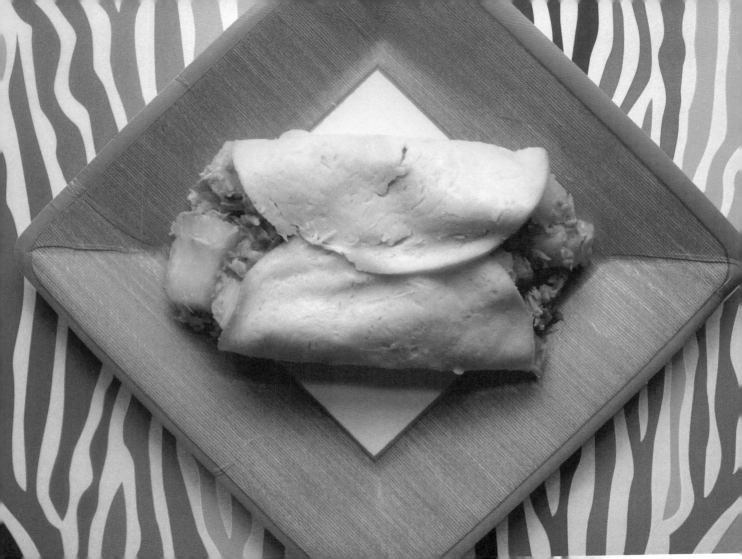

APPLE BACON TURKEY WRAP

Ingredients

* 5 Bacon Slices, Cooked
* 1 Small Apple, Diced
* 1 Thick Cut Slice of Turkey

Directions

1. Stuff turkey slice with bacon and diced apple.

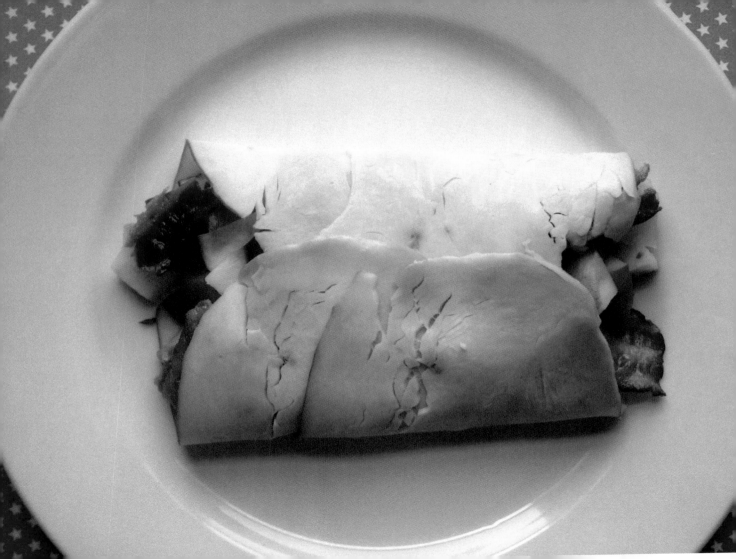

SWEET HOT PEACHES TURKEY WRAP

Ingredients

* 1 Peach, Diced
* 1 Tablespoon Maple Syrup
* 2 Tablespoons Walnuts
* Thick Cut Slice of Turkey

Directions

1. Heat the peaches on a pan over medium heat until soft.

2. Stuff the turkey slice with peaches. Top with walnuts and drizzle with maple syrup.

17

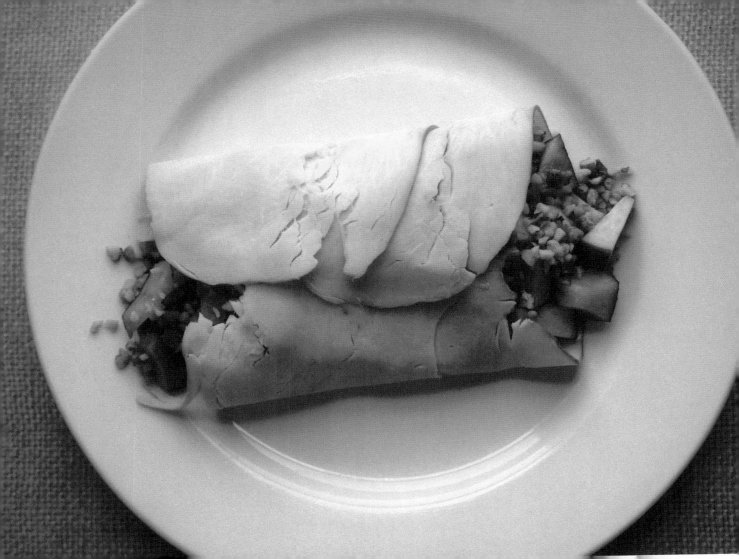

BACON ASPARAGUS TURKEY WRAP

Ingredients

* 3 Bacon Slices, Cooked
* 1 Teaspoon Olive Oil
* 4-6 Asparagus Spears
* 1/3 Cup Broccoli Florets
* 1 Tablespoon Shallots
* Thick Cut Slice of Turkey

Directions

1. Heat the oil, asparagus, broccoli, and shallots over medium heat until soft.

2. Stuff the turkey slice with bacon and hot vegetables.

19

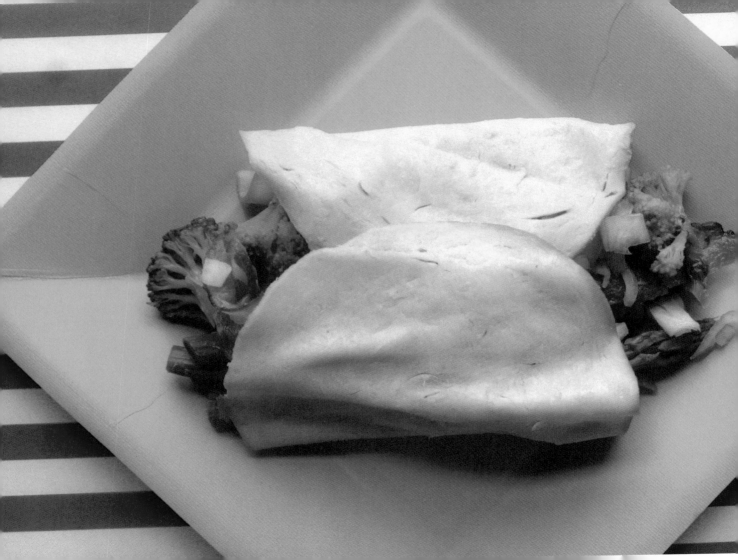

STRAWBERRY COCONUT TURKEY WRAP

Ingredients

* 1 Cup Strawberries, Sliced
* 2 Tablespoons Coconut Flakes
* 1/3 Cup Baby Spinach Leaves
* Thick Cut Slice of Turkey

Directions

1. Stuff the turkey slice with strawberries, coconut flakes, and baby spinach leaves.

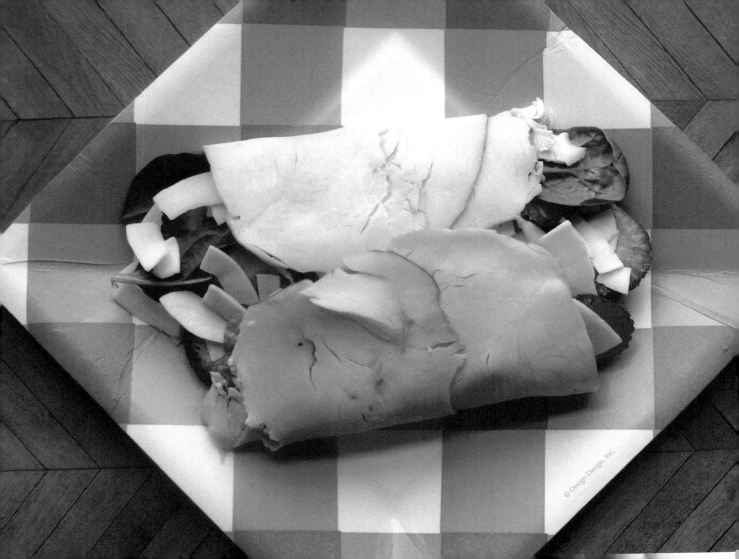

BACON, EGG, & GUACAMOLE TURKEY WRAP

Ingredients

* 1 Large Egg
* 1/2 Teaspoon Olive Oil
* Salt & Pepper to Taste
* 4 Bacon Slices, Cooked
* 2 Tablespoons Guacamole
* Thick Cut Slice of Turkey

Directions

1. Heat the oil and egg over medium heat until cooked through. Add salt and pepper to taste.

2. Crumble the bacon and sprinkle into the eggs.

3. Stuff the turkey slice with eggs, bacon, and guacamole.

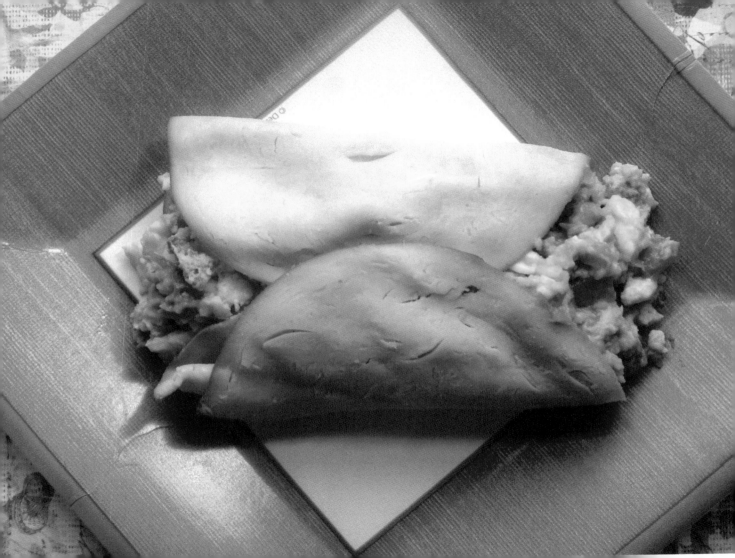

SPINACH SCRAMBLED EGGS TURKEY WRAP

Ingredients

* 1 Large Egg
* 1/2 Teaspoon Olive Oil
* Salt and Pepper to Taste
* 1/2 Cup Fresh Spinach
* 1/3 Cup Mushrooms, Sliced
* 1 Tablespoon Salsa
* Thick Cut Slice of Turkey

Directions

1. Scramble the eggs, olive oil, mushrooms, spinach, and salsa together and heat over medium heat until cooked through. Add salt and pepper to taste.

2. Stuff the turkey slice with spinach scrambled eggs.

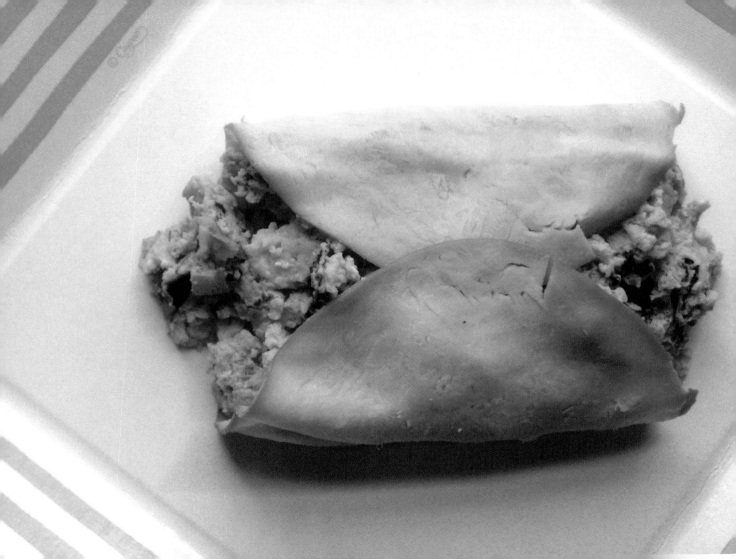

BEEF NACHO TURKEY WRAP

Ingredients

* 1/2 Cup Ground Beef, Cooked
* 3 Tablespoons Beef Broth
* 2 Tablespoons Black Olives, Sliced
* 6 Jalapeno Slices
* 1/3 Avocado, Diced
* 1/3 Cup Romaine Lettuce
* Thick Cut Slice of Turkey

Directions

1. Heat the beef broth, ground beef, olives, and jalapenos over medium heat until hot.

2. Stuff the turkey slice with beef mixture, romaine lettuce, and avocado.

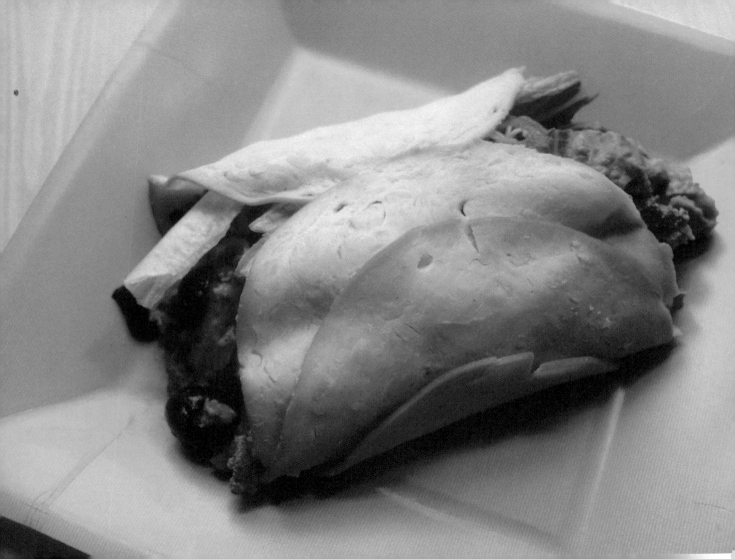

SALMON SALAD TURKEY WRAP

Ingredients

* 1/2 Can Salmon
* 1 Tablespoon Coconut Milk
* 1/2 Teaspoon Lemon Pepper
* 2 Tablespoons Shallots
* 1/4 Cup Cucumber, Sliced
* 1 Hard Boiled Egg, Diced
* 2 Bacon Slices, Crumbled
* Thick Cut Slice of Turkey

Directions

1. Mix all ingredients, except turkey, in a bowl to make salmon salad.

2. Stuff the turkey slice with salmon salad.

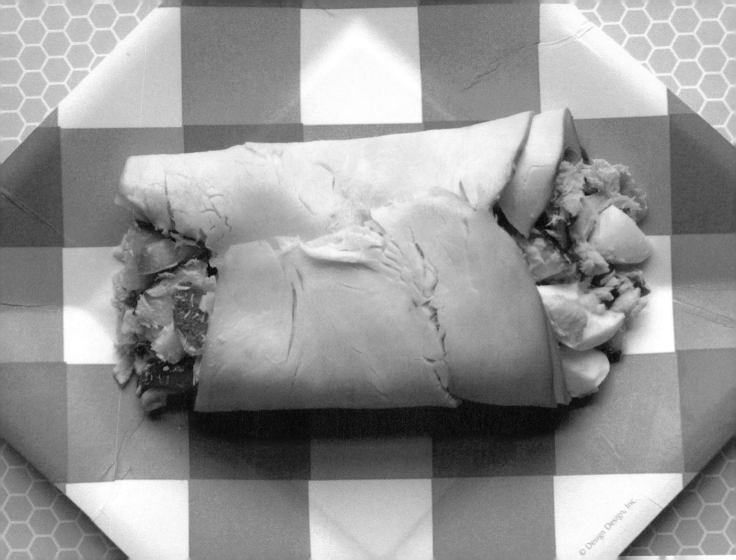

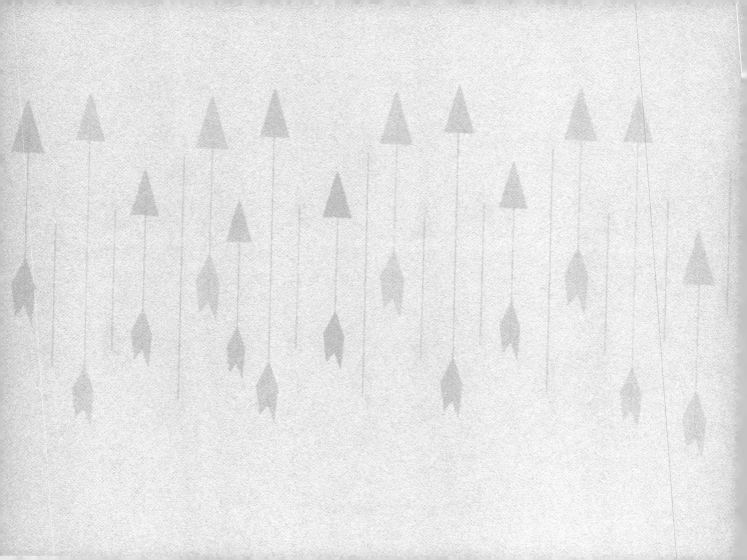

HAM

HAWAiiAN COCONUTTY HAM WRAP

Ingredients

* 1/4 Cup Coconut Flakes
* 1/2 Cup Pineapple, Diced
* Thick Cut Slice of
  Ham

Directions

1. Heat the ham slice on pan or over a panini grill.

2. Stuff the ham slice with pineapple chunks and coconut flakes.

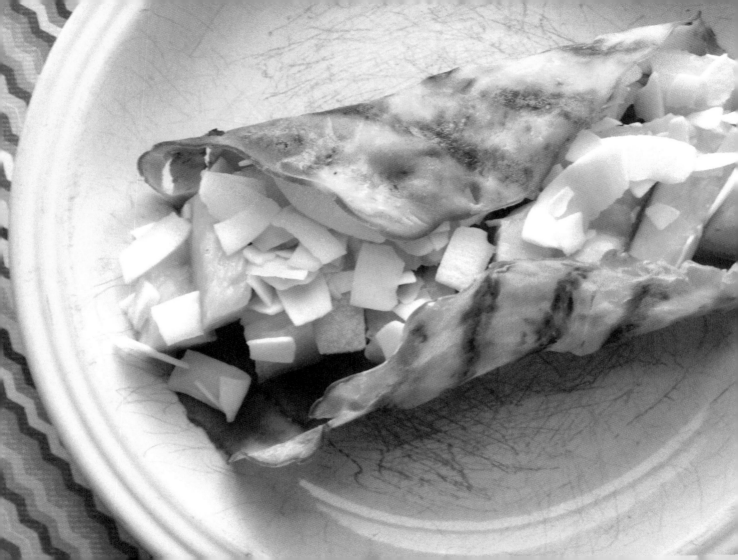

BACON, EGG, & GUACAMOLE HAM WRAP

Ingredients

* 4 Bacon Slices
* 3 Tablespoons Guacamole
* 1 Hard Boiled Egg, Sliced
* 1/2 Cup Cucumber, Sliced
* Thick Cut Slice of Ham

Directions

1. Heat ham slice on pan or over a panini grill.

2. Stuff ham slice with bacon, guacamole, hard boiled egg, and cucumber.

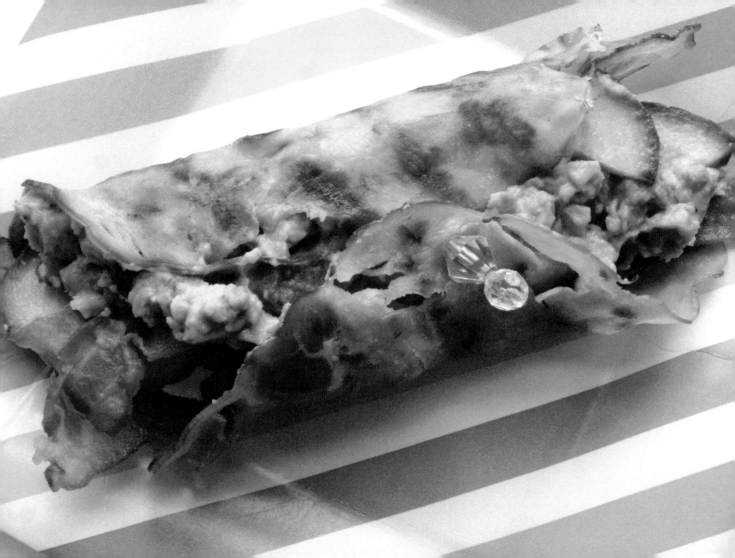

HONEY BANANA NUT HAM WRAP

Ingredients

* 1 Banana, Sliced
* 1 Teaspoon Honey
* 1 Tablespoon Walnuts
* 1 Tablespoon Macadamia Nuts
* Thick Cut Slice of
   Ham

Directions

1. Heat the ham slice and banana slices on pan or over a panini grill.

2. Stuff the ham slice with bananas. Drizzle with honey and top with nuts.

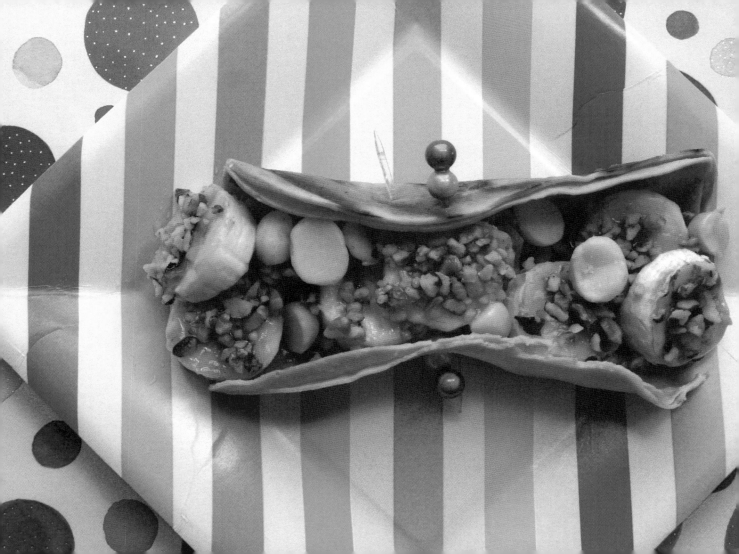

SMASHED BLACKBERRY HAM WRAP

Ingredients

* 1/2 Cup Blackberries
* 1/4 Cup Walnuts
* 1/3 Cup Arugula
* Thick Cut Slice of Ham

Directions

1. Smash blackberries in a small bowl using a fork.

2. Stuff the ham slice with smashed blackberries and top with nuts and arugula.

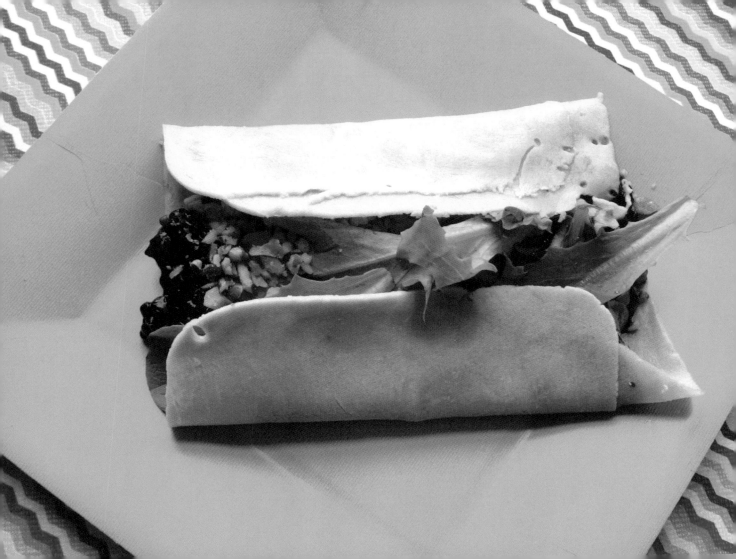

MAPLE BACON & EGG HAM WRAP

Ingredients

* 1 Teaspoon Olive Oil
* 2 Eggs
* 2 Bacon Slices, Crumbled
* 1 Tablespoon Maple Syrup
* Thick Cut Slice of Ham

Directions

1. Heat and stir the oil, eggs, maple syrup, and bacon over medium heat until eggs are cooked through.

2. Heat the ham slice on pan or over a panini grill.

3. Stuff the ham slice with hot bacon and egg mixture.

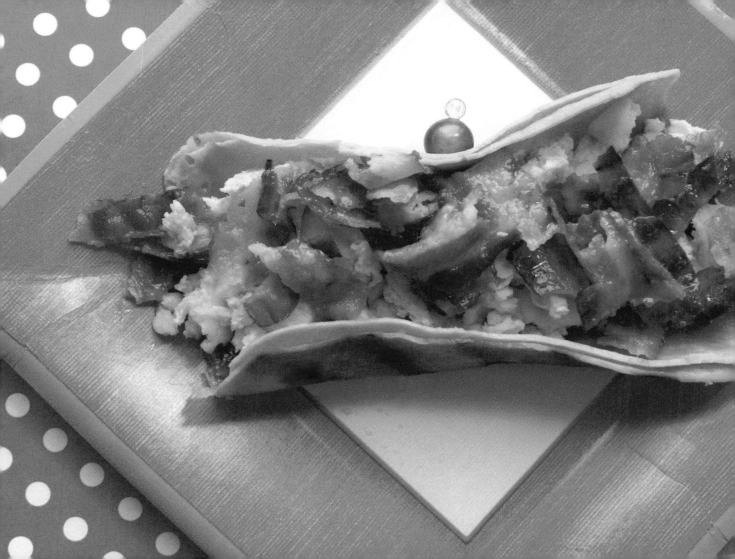

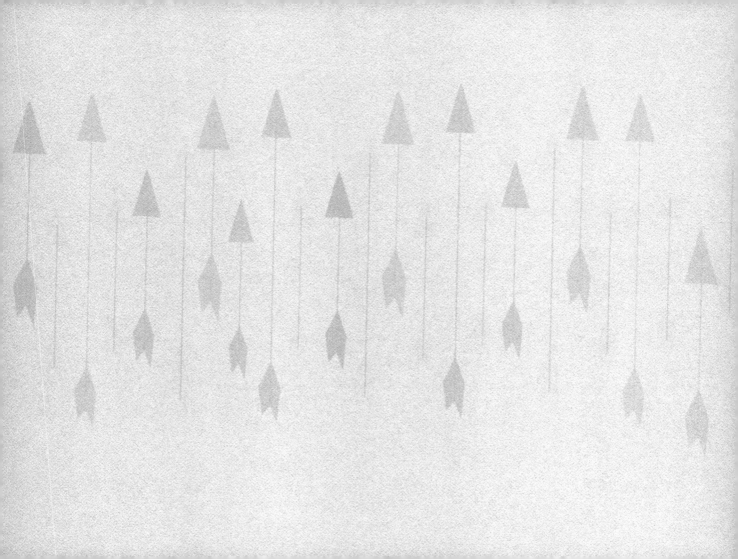

LETTUCE

FIESTA CHICKEN LETTUCE WRAP

Ingredients

* 2 Slices Thin Cut Chicken Breast, Thawed
* 1 Teaspoon Olive Oil
* Salt & Pepper to Taste
* 1/2 Small Avocado, Diced
* 1/2 Small Lime
* 1/3 Cup Tomato or Salsa
* 1-2 Large Romaine Lettuce Leaves

Directions

1. Heat the chicken and oil over medium heat until cooked through. Season with salt and pepper to taste.

2. Stuff the lettuce with chicken breast, avocado, and tomato or salsa. Squeeze lime juice over the top.

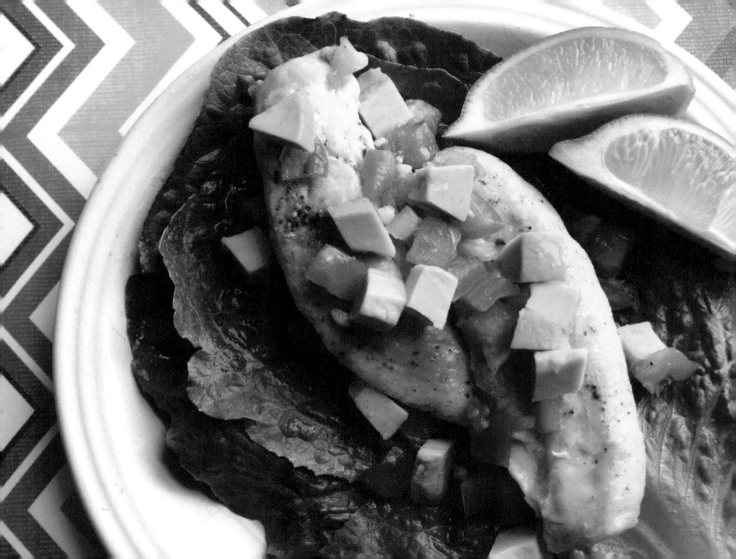

ZESTY BACON & EGG LETTUCE WRAP

Ingredients

*4 Bacon Slices, Cooked
* 1 Hard Boiled Egg, Sliced
* 1/4 Cup Salsa
* 1-2 Large Romaine Lettuce Leaves

Directions

1. Stuff the lettuce leaves with bacon, eggs, and salsa.

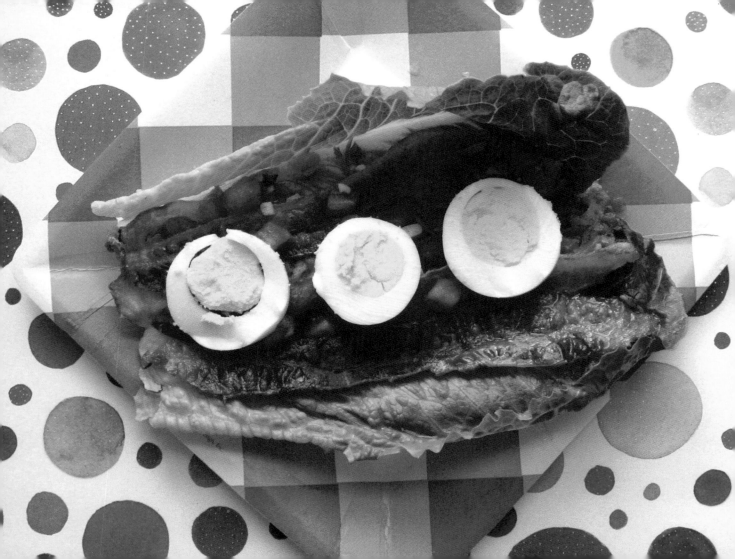

PEACHY SALMON BACON LETTUCE WRAP

Ingredients

* 1/2 Cup Smoked Salmon
* 2-3 Bacon Slices, Cooked
*1/2 Cup Peaches, Diced
* 1-2 Large Romaine Lettuce Leaves

Directions

1. Heat the smoked salmon on a non-stick pan for 3-4 minutes.

2. Stuff lettuce leaves with smoked salmon, bacon slices, and peaches.

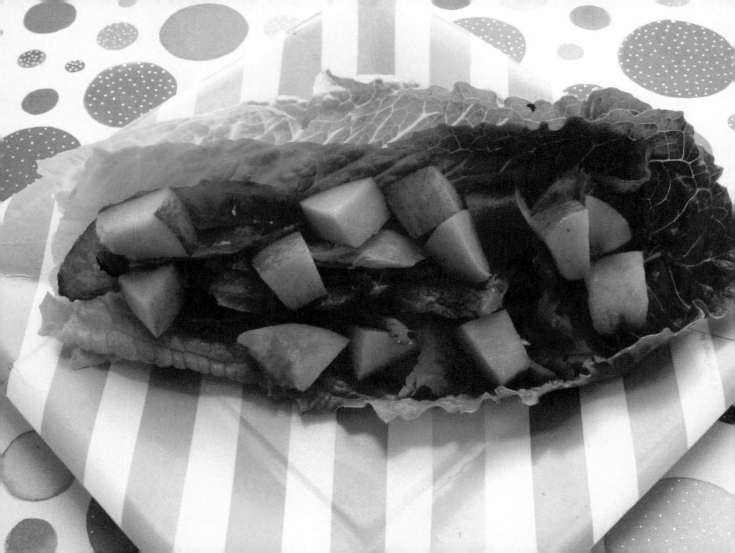

RISE & SHINE SALMON LETTUCE WRAP

Ingredients

* 1/2 Cup Smoked Salmon
* 1 Large Egg
* 1 Teaspoon Olive Oil
* Salt & Pepper to Taste
* 1/2 Avocado, Diced
* 1-2 Large Romaine Lettuce Leaves

Directions

1. Heat the oil, salmon, and eggs over medium heat until the eggs are cooked through. Add salt and pepper to taste.

2. Stuff the lettuce leaves with eggs and salmon. Top with diced avocado.

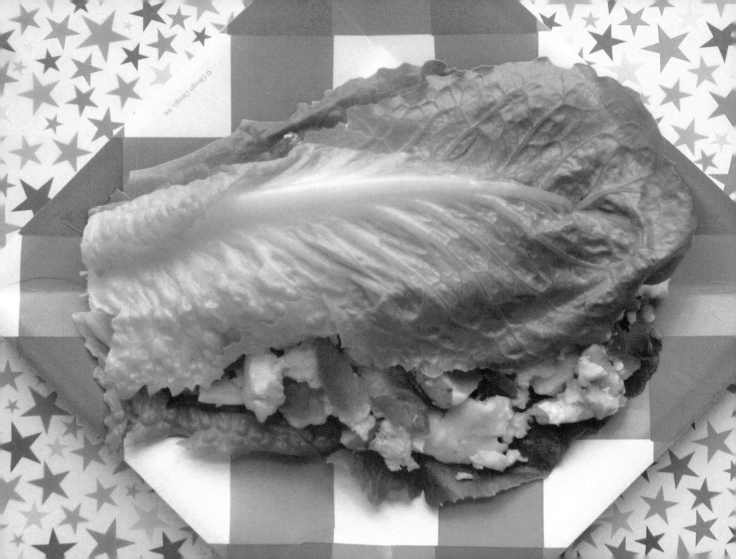

GUACAMOLE SALMON CAKE LETTUCE WRAP

Ingredients

* 1 Can Salmon
* 1 Egg
* Salt & Pepper to Taste
* 3 Tablespoons Guacamole
* 1/2 Lime
* 1/3 Cup Cabbage
* 1-2 Large Romaine Lettuce Leaves

Directions

1. Mix the salmon, eggs, salt, and pepper in a bowl. Form mixture into 2 patties.

2. Heat the oil over medium heat until the pan is hot. Heat salmon patties for 6-7 minutes.

3. Stuff the lettuce leaves with salmon patties, guacamole, and cabbage. Squeeze lime juice over the top.

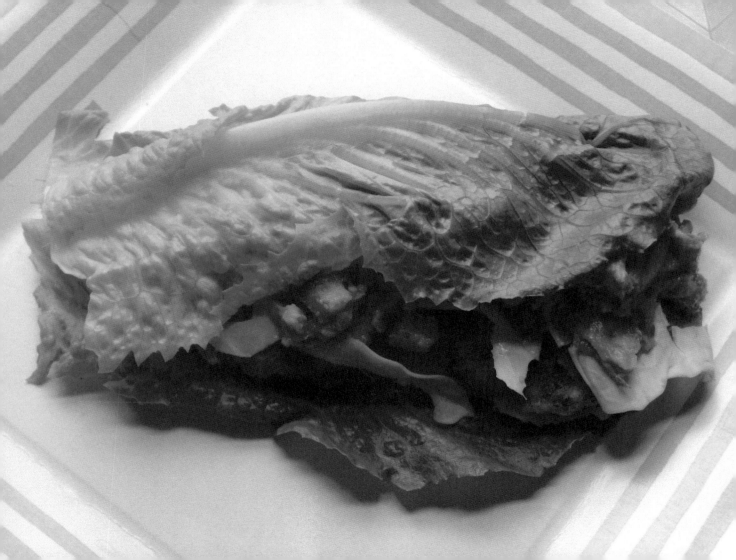

MANGO HADDOCK LETTUCE WRAP

Ingredients

* 1/3 Cup Mango, Diced
* 1/3 Cup Pineapple, Diced
* 1/3 Cup Peaches, Diced
* 1 Small Haddock Fillet
* 1-2 Large Romaine Lettuce Leaves

Directions

1. Preheat oven to 450 degrees.

2. Place haddock on baking sheet and cook for 15 minutes or until it flakes easily.

3. Stuff the lettuce leaves with haddock and fruit.

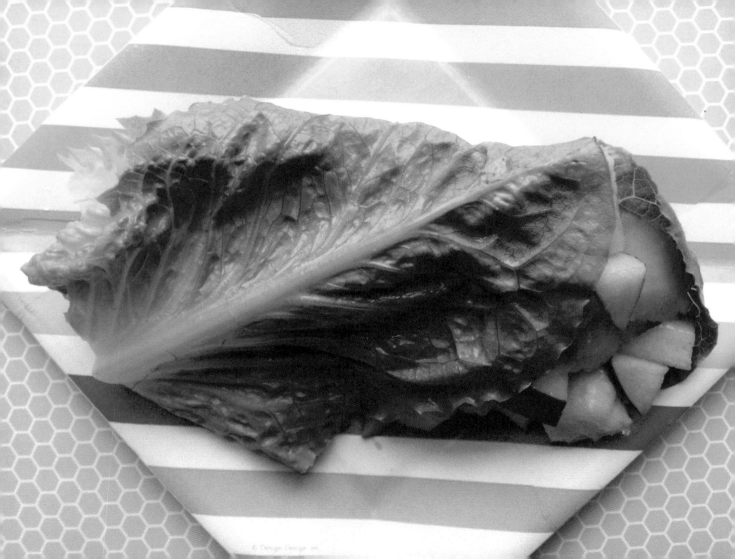

ZINGY EGG SALAD LETTUCE WRAP

Ingredients

* 3 Hard Boiled Eggs
* 1 Tablespoon Mustard
* 1 Tablespoon Dijon Mustard
* 2 Tablespoons Shallots
* 2 Bacon Slices, Crumbled
* 1-2 Large Romaine Lettuce Leaves

Directions

1. Mix all ingredients, excluding lettuce leaves, in a bowl to make zingy egg salad.

2. Stuff lettuce leaves with egg salad.

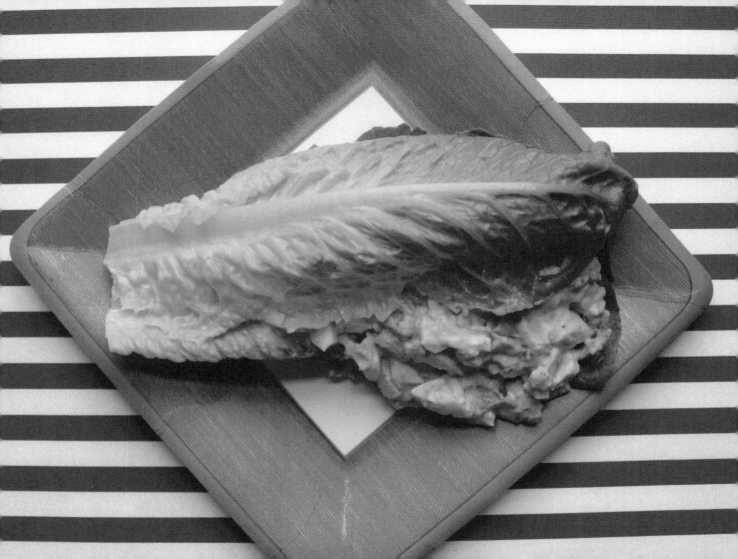

JALAPENO BEEF LETTUCE WRAP

Ingredients

* 1/3 lb. Ground Beef, Thawed
* 2 Baby Bella Mushrooms, Sliced
* 10 Jalapeno Slices
* 2 Tablespoons Onions, Chopped
* 1/4 Cup Tomatoes, Chopped
* 4 Tablespoons Beef Broth
* 1-2 Large Romaine Lettuce Leaves

Directions

1. Heat the ground beef and beef broth over medium heat until almost cooked through.

2. Add the mushrooms, jalapenos, onions, and tomatoes to the beef. Cover and cook for an additional 4 minutes.

3. Stuff the lettuce leaves with the beef mixture.

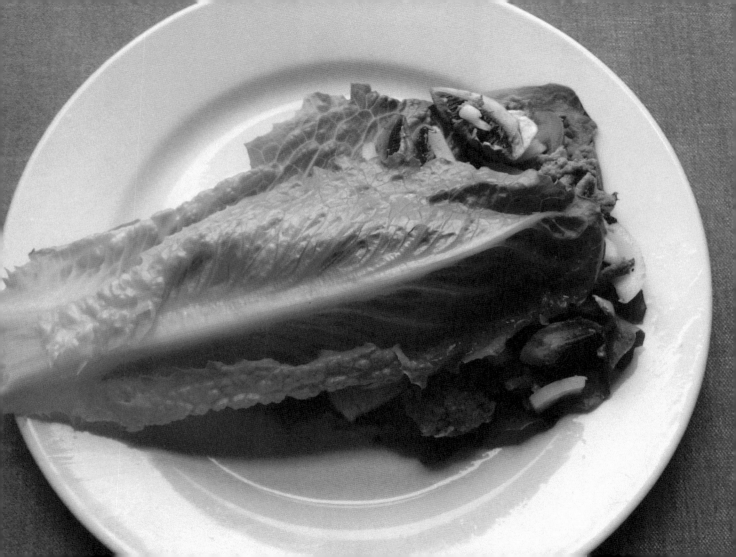

BEEF & BROCCOLI LETTUCE WRAP

Ingredients

* 1/3 lb. Ground Beef
* 4 Tablespoons Beef Broth
* 1/2 Cup Broccoli Florets
* 1-2 Large Romaine Lettuce Leaves

Directions

1. Heat the ground beef and beef broth over medium heat until almost cooked through.

2. Add the broccoli florets to the beef. Cover and cook for an additional 4 minutes.

3. Stuff the lettuce leaves with the beef and broccoli.

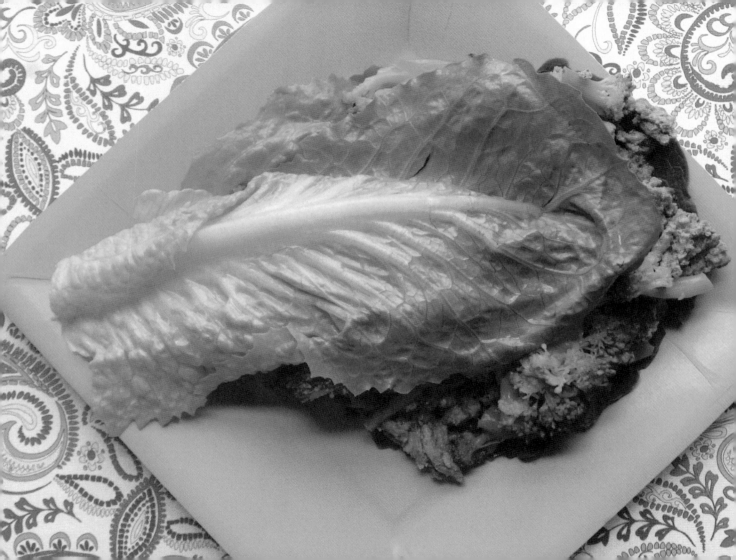

SPICY LIME CHICKEN LETTUCE WRAP

Ingredients

* 2 Slices Thin Cut Chicken, Thawed
* 1 Teaspoon Olive Oil
* Salt & Pepper to Taste
* 4-6 Jalapeno Slices
* 1/2 Small Lime
* 3 Tablespoons Salsa
*1-2 Large Romaine Lettuce Leaves

Directions

1. Heat the olive oil and chicken over medium heat until cooked through. Squeeze lime juice over hot chicken. Add salt and pepper to taste.

2. Stuff lettuce leaves with chicken, jalapenos, and salsa.

63

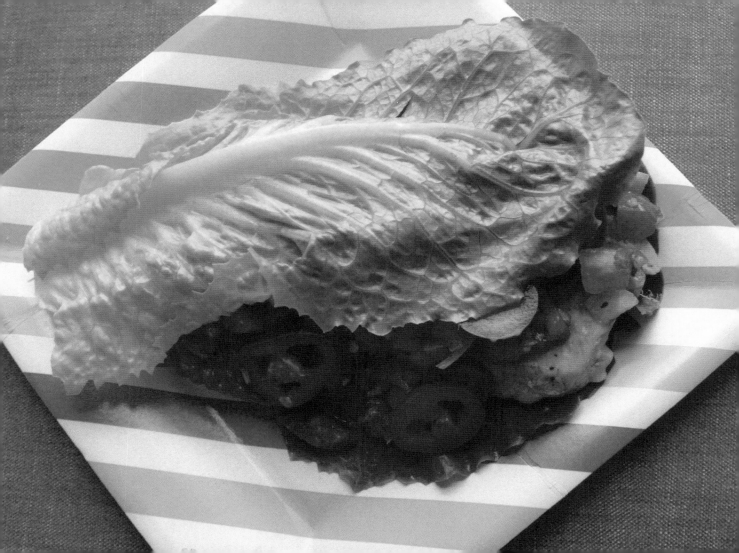

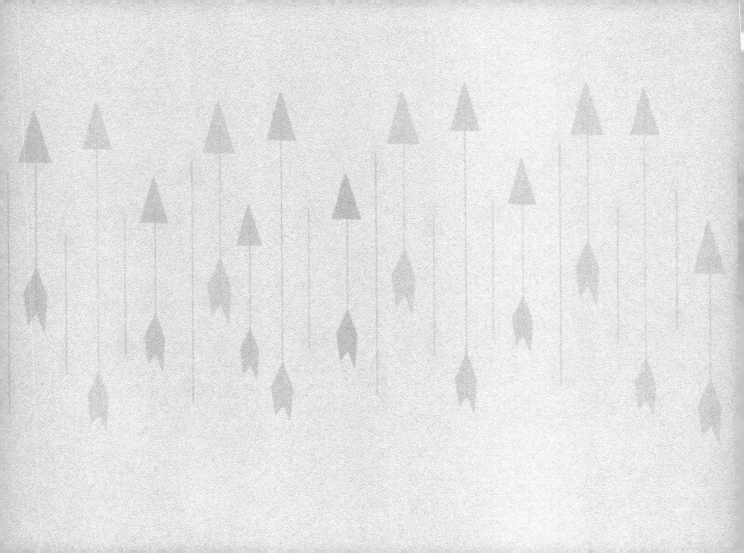

SALMON

TROPICAL CRAB SALAD SALMON WRAP

Ingredients

* 1 Tablespoon Coconut Milk
* 1/2 Can Crab Meat
* 1 Tablespoon Shallots
* 1 Tablespoon Jalapeno, Chopped
* 1 Teaspoon Lime Juice
* 1/4 Cup Baby Spinach
* 3-4 Cucumber Slices
* 1/3 Cup Pineapple, Diced
* Thick Slice of Smoked Salmon

Directions

1. Mix all ingredients, excluding smoked salmon, in a bowl.

2. Stuff the smoked salmon with crab salad.

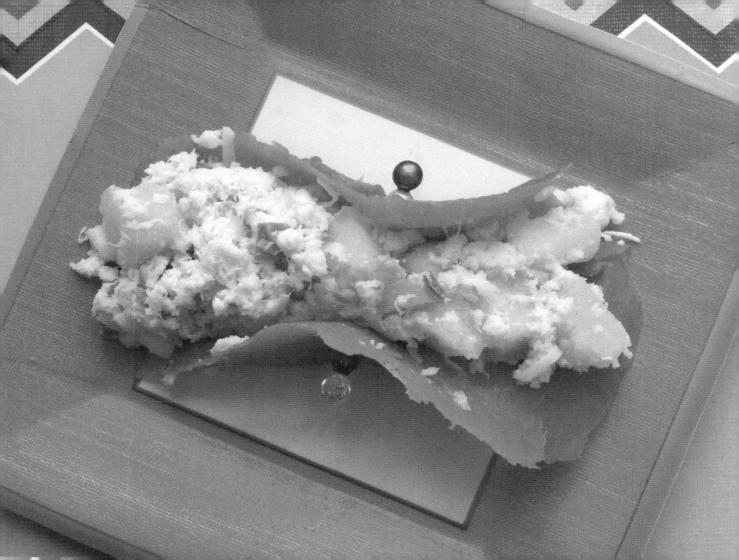

FRUITY NUTTY SALMON WRAP

Ingredients

* 1/4 Cup Cashews
* 1 Nectarine, Diced
* Thick Slice of Smoked Salmon

Directions

1. Stuff the smoked salmon slice with diced nectarine and cashews.

69

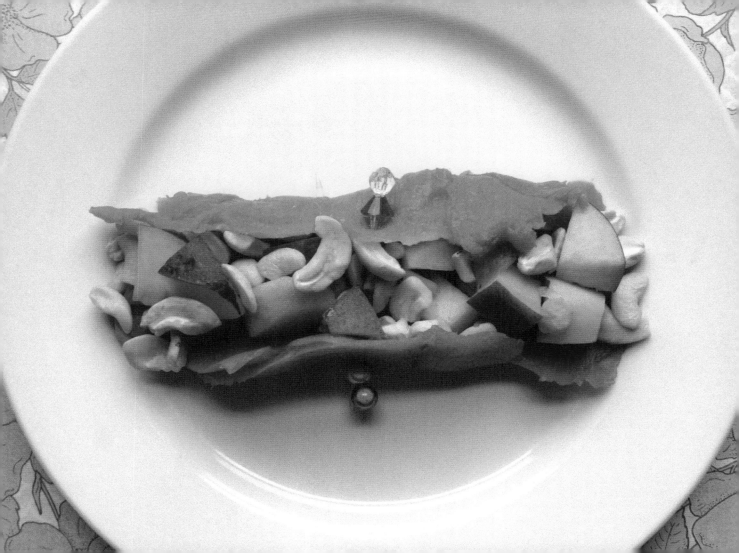

CHUNKY PINEAPPLE SALMON WRAP

Ingredients

* 1 Cup Pineapple Chunks
* 1/4 Cup Coconut Flakes
* Thick Slice of Smoked Salmon

Directions

1. Stuff the smoked salmon slice with pineapple chunks and top with coconut flakes.

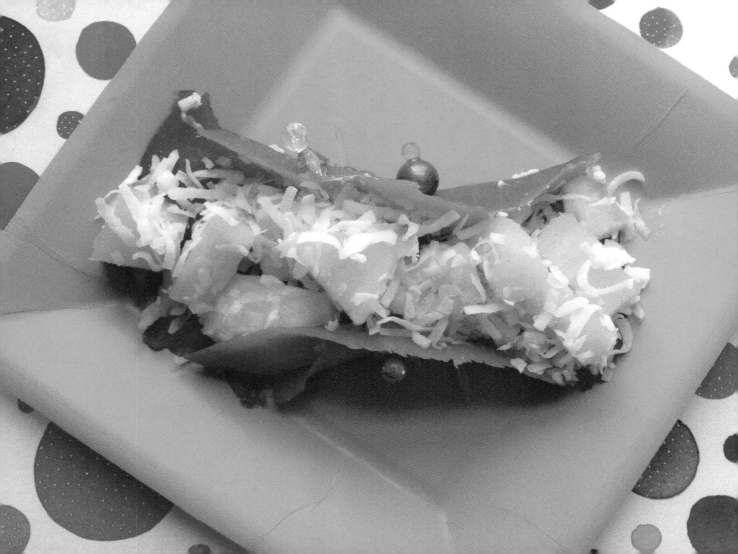

SHRiMPY BACON SALMON WRAP

Ingredients

* 4 Bacon Slices, Cooked
* 1/2 Cup Shrimp, Thawed
* 1/2 Avocado, Diced
* 6-8 Baby Spinach Leaves
* Thick Slice of Smoked Salmon

Directions

1. Stuff the salmon slice with bacon, shrimp, avocado, and spinach.

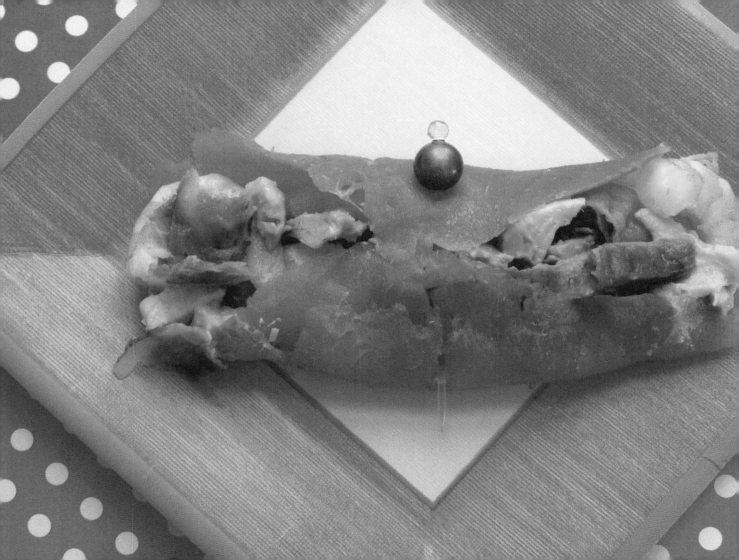

CREAMY CRUNCHY BACON SALMON WRAP

Ingredients

* 4 Bacon Slices, Cooked
* 1/2 Cup Cucumber, Sliced
* 1/2 Avocado, Diced
* Thick Slice of Smoked Salmon

Directions

1. Stuff smoked salmon slice with bacon, cucumber, and avocado.

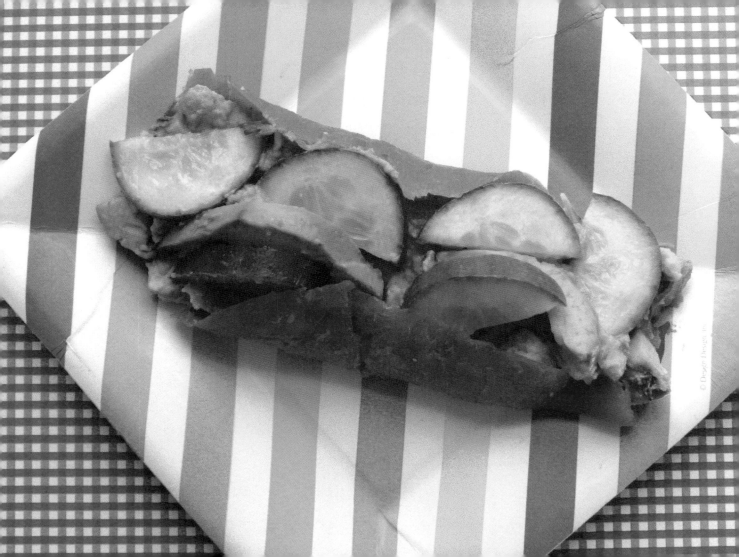

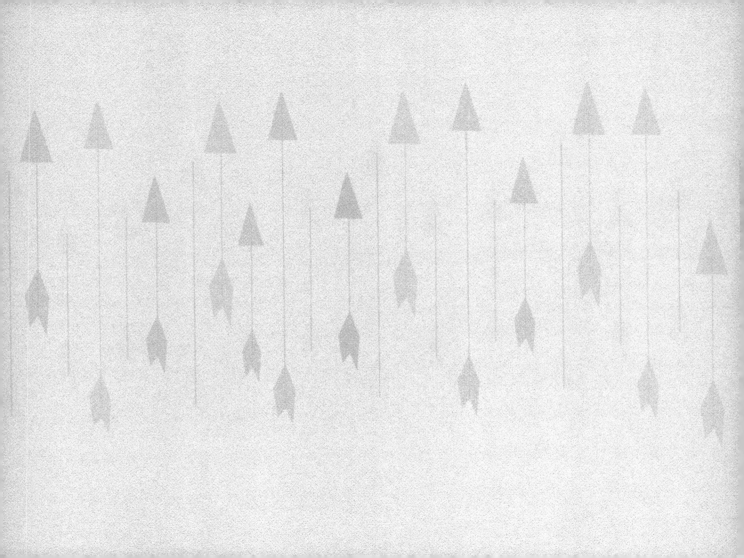

CHiCKEN

JUiCY PEPPER & ONiON CHiCKEN WRAP

Ingredients

* 1/2 Green Pepper, Sliced
* 1/2 Red Pepper, Sliced
* 6 Jalapeno Slices
* Thick Cut Slice of Lemon Pepper Chicken

Directions

1. Heat the green pepper, red pepper, and jalapeno slices over medium heat until soft.

2. Heat the lemon pepper chicken slice on pan or over a panini grill.

3. Stuff the lemon pepper chicken slice with peppers.

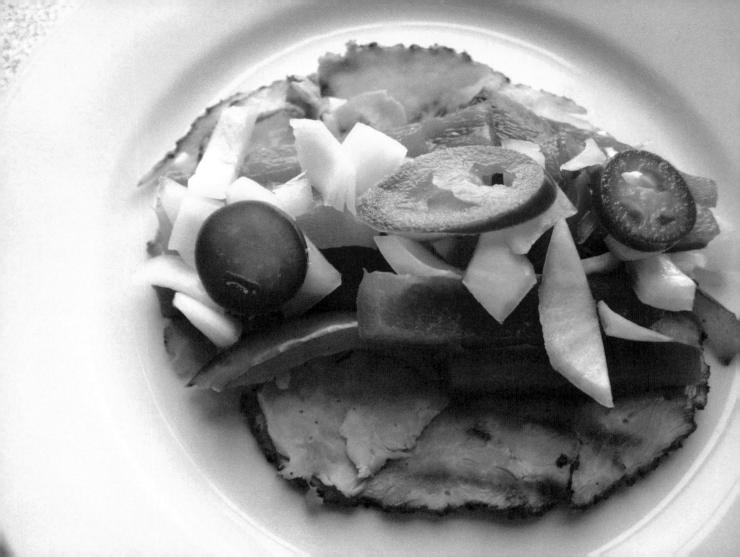

CITRUSY BACON CHICKEN WRAP

Ingredients

* 3-4 Slices Cooked Bacon
* 1/2 Small Lemon
* 1/2 Small Lime
* 1/4 Cup Romaine Lettuce
* Thick Cut Slice of Lemon Pepper Chicken

Directions

1. Heat the lemon pepper chicken slice on pan or over a panini grill.

2. Stuff lemon pepper chicken slice with lettuce and bacon.

3. Squeeze lemon and lime juice over lettuce and bacon.

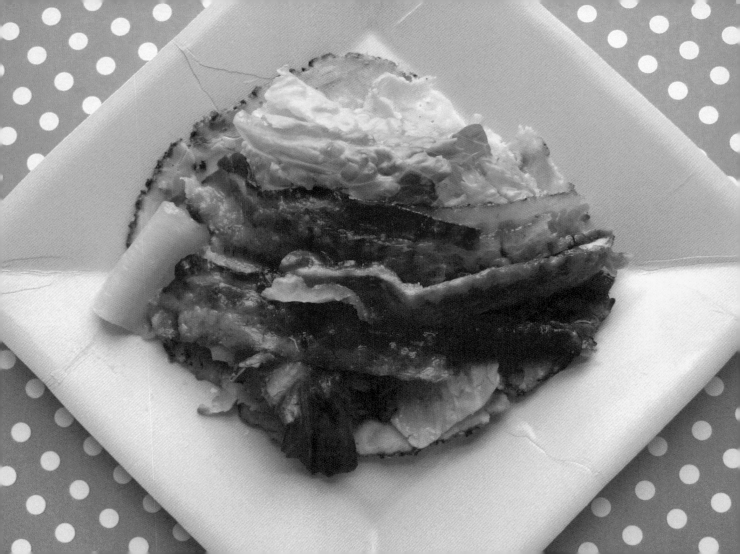

ZiPPY AVOCADO CHICKEN WRAP

Ingredients

* 1/2 Diced Avocado
* 1/4 Cup Chopped Shallots
* 1 Slice Ham
* Thick Cut Slice of
Lemon Pepper Chicken

Directions

1. Heat the lemon pepper chicken slice on pan or over a panini grill.

2. Stuff a slice of ham with diced avocado and shallots.

3. Roll up the stuffed ham slice and place it in the lemon pepper chicken slice.

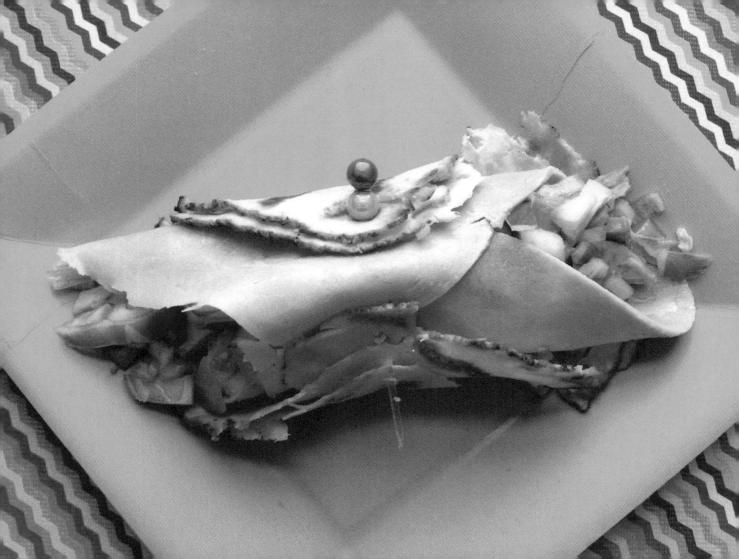

KiCKiN' LEMON MUSHROOM CHICKEN WRAP

Ingredients

* 1/2 Small Lemon
* 1/3 Red Bell Pepper, Sliced
* 1/3 Green Bell Pepper, Sliced
* 1/3 Yellow Bell Pepper, Sliced
* 1/4 Cup Cucumber, Sliced
* 2 Baby Bella Mushrooms, Sliced
* Thick Cut Slice of
Lemon Pepper Chicken

Directions

1. Heat the peppers over medium heat until soft.

2. Stuff the lemon pepper chicken slice with peppers, cucumber, and mushrooms.

3. Squeeze lemon juice over peppers, cucumbers, and mushrooms.

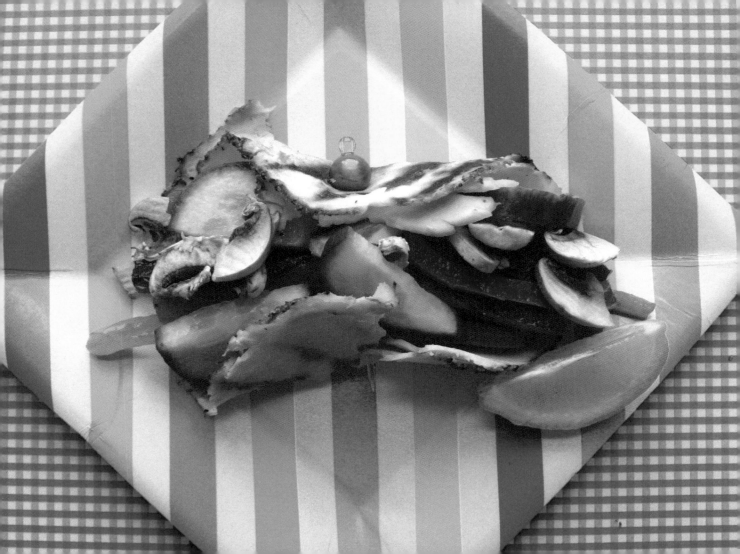

SUSHI STYLE CHICKEN WRAP

Ingredients

* 1/3 Cup Thawed Shrimp
* 1/2 Avocado, Diced
* 1/3 Cup Grilled Chicken, Diced
* 1/4 Cup Cucumber, Sliced
* 1/4 Cup Shredded Carrots
* Thick Cut Slice of
Lemon Pepper Chicken

Directions

1. Heat cooked grilled chicken over medium heat until warm.

2. Stuff a cold lemon pepper chicken slice with shrimp, avocado, cucumber, carrots, and grilled chicken.

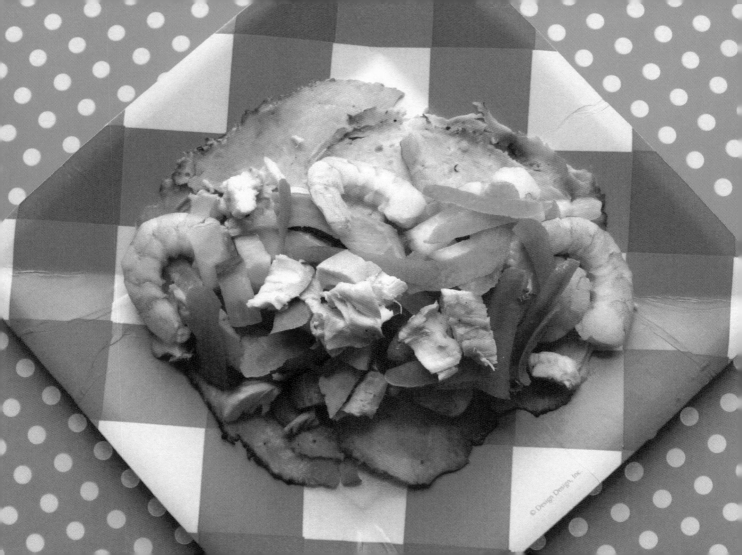

NUTTY ORANGE HONEY CHICKEN WRAP

Ingredients

* 1/3 Cup Walnuts
* 1 Tablespoon Honey
* 1/4 Orange Slice
* 1-2 Slices of Thawed Thin Cut Chicken Breast
* 1 Teaspoon Olive Oil
* 6-8 Baby Spinach Leaves
* Thick Cut Slice of Lemon Pepper Chicken

Directions

1. Heat the lemon pepper chicken slice on pan or over a panini grill.

2. Heat the olive oil and thin cut chicken breast over medium heat until cooked through.

3. Drizzle honey and juice from the orange slice over chicken. Cook for an additional 2 minutes.

4. Stuff the lemon pepper chicken slice with chicken breast and baby spinach leaves. Top with walnuts.

89

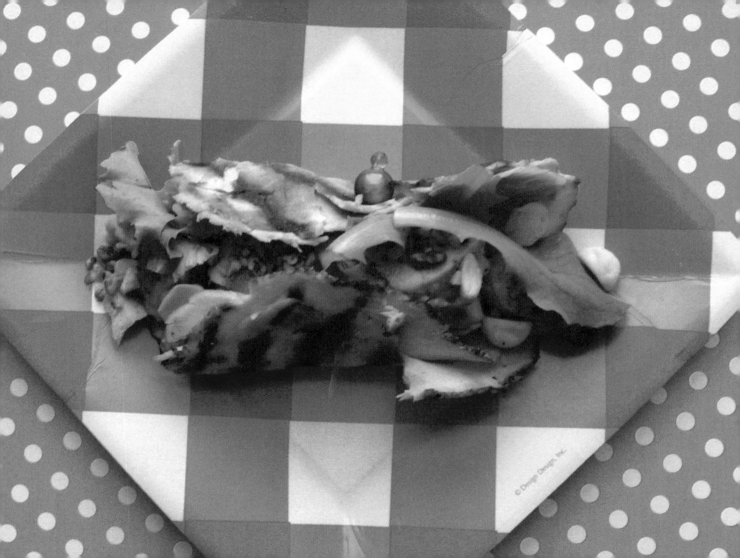

© Design Design, Inc.

CHICKEN POT PIE CHICKEN WRAP

Ingredients

* 2 Tablespoons Chicken Broth
* 1-2 Slices of Thawed Thin Cut Chicken Breast
* 1/4 Cup Peas
* 1/4 Cup Shredded Carrots
* 1 Baby Bella Mushroom, Sliced
* Thick Cut Slice of Lemon Pepper Chicken

Directions

1. Heat the lemon pepper chicken slice on pan or over a panini grill.

2. Heat 2 tablespoons of chicken broth and the thin cut chicken breast slices over medium heat until cooked through.

3. Add 1 tablespoon of chicken broth, along with the peas, carrots, and mushrooms to the pan and cook for an additional 4 minutes.

4. Stuff the lemon pepper chicken slice with chicken, peas, mushrooms, and carrots.

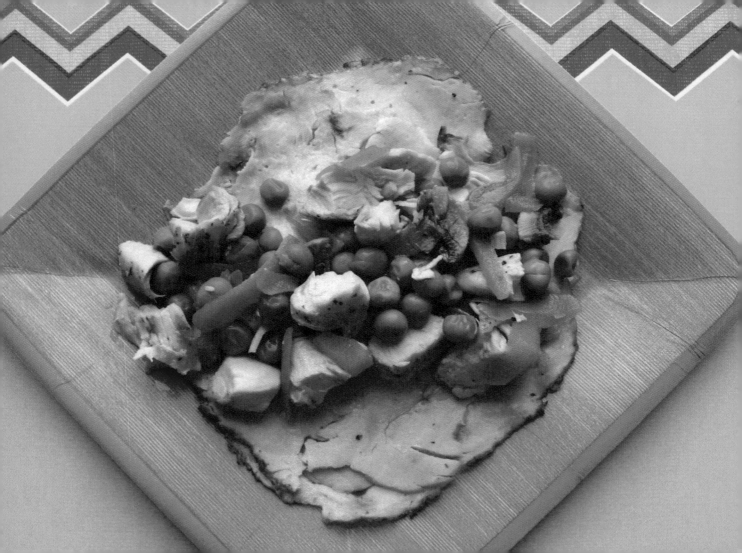

BEEFY BACON NACHO CHICKEN WRAP

Ingredients

* 1/3 lb. Ground Beef, Thawed
* 1 Tablespoon Olive Oil
* 2 Bacon Slices, Crumbled
* 6 Jalapeno Slices
* 3 Tablespoons Guacamole
* 2 Tablespoons Sliced Black Olives
* Thick Cut Slice of
Lemon Pepper Chicken

Directions

1. Heat the ground beef over medium heat with olive oil until cooked through.

2. Heat the lemon pepper chicken slice on pan or over a panini grill.

3. Stuff the lemon pepper chicken slice with beef, olives, bacon crumbles, guacamole, and jalapenos.

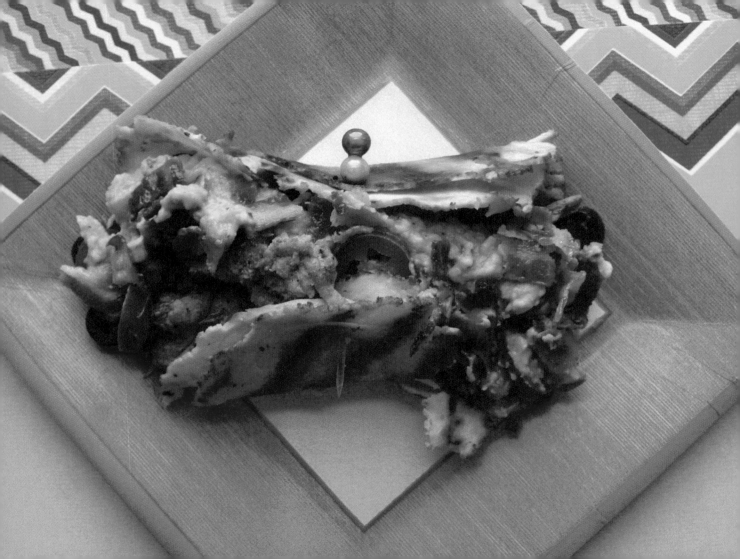

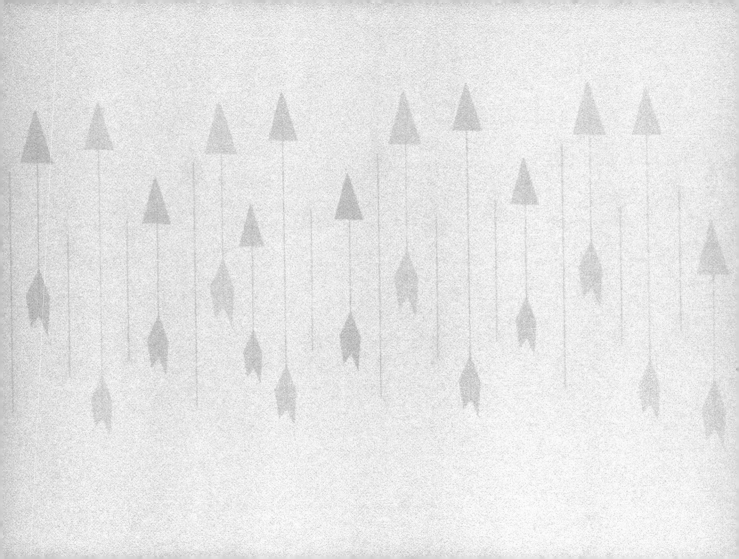

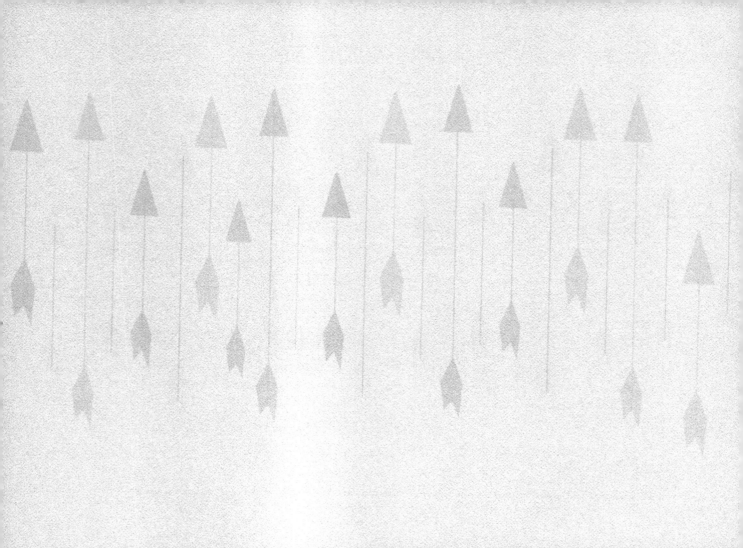

38367757R10058

Made in the USA
Lexington, KY
05 January 2015